This bite-sized boo
useful overview of
you to:

- Understand the in
wellbeing
- Improve the quality of your physical and mental health
- Reduce stress build up through a range of activities
- Enhance concentration levels and sharpen your memory
- Get moving and feel more flexible and energised

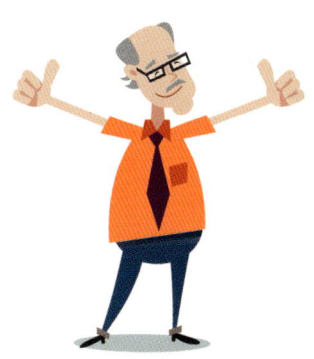

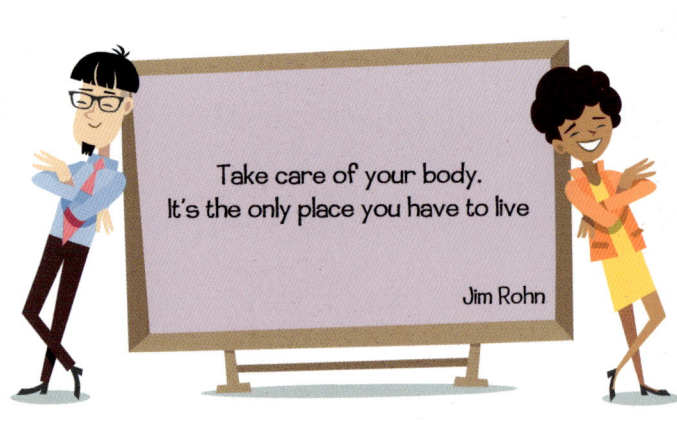

Movement

When we get moving, it can improve the quality of our lives, and movement is one of the most valuable things that we can do for our overall wellbeing. As human beings we have a basic psychological and physical need to move our bodies and it is helpful that we do this on a regular basis if we want to stay fit and well. This is especially important as we get older.

When we get active and move about it helps to improve our brain health, manage our weight, reduce our risk of disease and strengthen our bones and muscles. Low levels of movement are attributed to numerous physical and mental health problems, so to fully enjoy and engage with life we need to get moving.

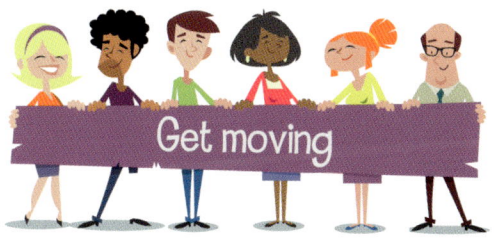

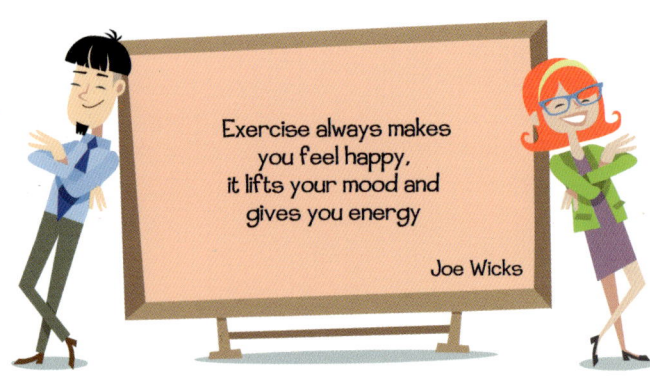

Movement and mood

Movement and exercise can improve our mental health by boosting our cognitive function and exercise has also been found to alleviate symptoms such as low self-esteem and social withdrawal. Moving about and getting some physical activity can reduce conditions such as depression and anxiety.

Exercise and movement can also reduce the levels of the body's stress hormones, such as adrenaline and cortisol, as well as stimulate the production of endorphins which are our feel-good hormones.

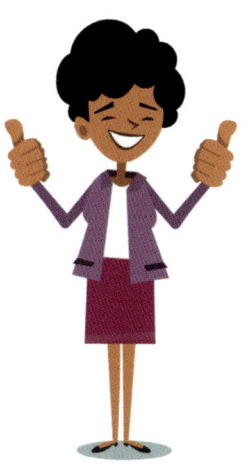

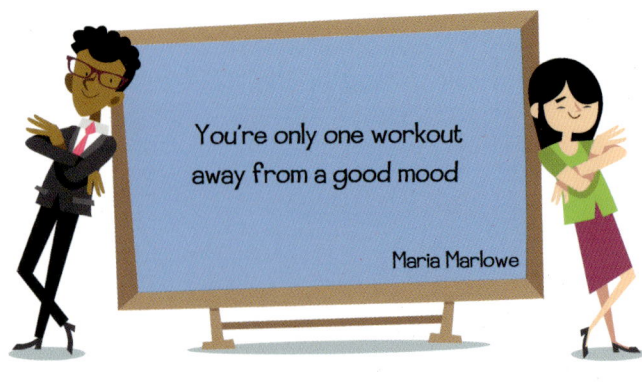

Movement and our brains

When we get moving and physically active it can promote the growth of neurons in our brains. This helps us to form new neural pathways which in turn will help our minds to be sharper and slow age-related decline. Hormones such as dopamine, norepinephrine and serotonin are also released which affects our focus and attention.

Whether we are going for a brisk walk or doing some simple stretches, movement can help reduce stress by allowing our brains to focus on other things such as our breathing and the rhythm of the movements. We will feel much better when we get active and it will help us to feel more focused and energised.

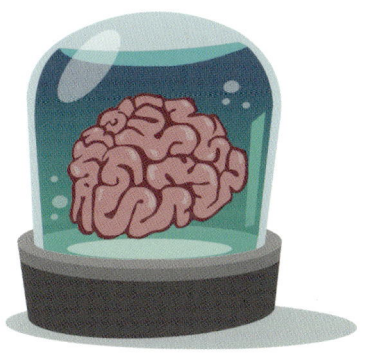

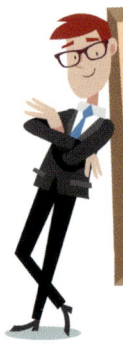

Motion is the lotion.
The more you move your body,
the more your joints are getting
the natural lubricants they need
to stay healthy and active

Dr Greg Ford

Movement and our bodies

Flexibility is the key to stability and a flexible body is agile and resilient. Movement causes our muscle fibres to contract and relax, maintaining the elasticity and power in the muscle. We need strong flexible muscles to help us with general activity and to prevent injury.

Movement and physical activity helps our bodies to maintain good joint and muscle mobility and it also helps us to promote bone, ligament and tendon strength. Motion is indeed the lotion because movement increases the circulation of blood and synovial fluid providing nutrients and lubrication to the joints. We can lose mobility and flexibility as we age. However, the good news is that it is something we can maintain and even improve when we keep moving.

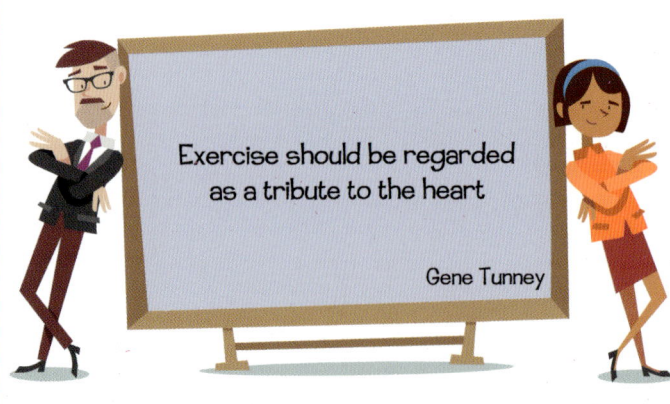

Movement and our hearts

Movement and physical activity can have a very positive impact on our heart health by helping to reduce our cholesterol and blood pressure, as well as boost our metabolism. Movement and exercise have also been shown to reduce the risk of many other diseases such as diabetes, stroke and certain cancers.

Movement and exercise also use up energy which burns calories, making it easier for us to manage our weight as well as support our cardiovascular function. The more consistently we move about and keep active, the greater the health benefits will be.

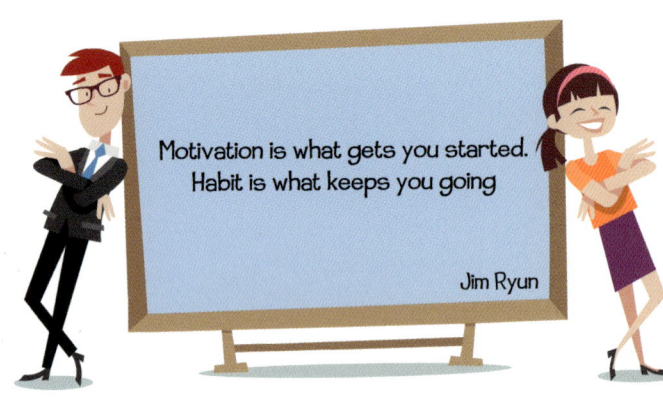

Get moving

There are many ways that we can get moving and one of the best ways is to make a conscious effort to move about as much as we can and build good habits.

It is the little things that we incorporate into our everyday life that will make a big difference. A gentle stretch first thing in the morning, taking the stairs instead of the lift, making sure we get more regular breaks from our desks, doing some stretches or squats whilst we watch TV, joining an exercise class or doing some housework can all have a positive impact.

So here are a few more suggestions of ways we can incorporate movement and activity into our everyday lives and get moving.

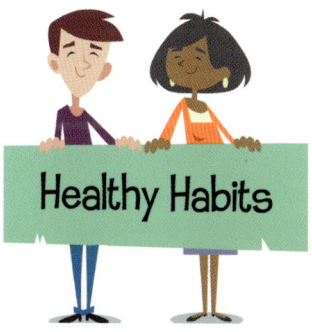

Get moving

Get walking

Walking is highly beneficial for our mental health and overall mood, and setting ourselves a daily step goal by tracking our steps is a great way to stay motivated. Here are a few ways to get those extra steps in:

- ✓ Make sure you get outside every day, no matter what the weather
- ✓ Use lunch breaks to go for an energising stroll
- ✓ Walk to the shops rather than take the car
- ✓ Use the stairs instead of the lift or escalator
- ✓ Join a walking group or get a walking buddy
- ✓ Get a dog or volunteer to walk someone else's
- ✓ Have a walking work meeting rather than sit at a computer
- ✓ Jog on the spot throughout the day
- ✓ Listen to podcasts and audiobooks when walking

NB – 10,000 steps is roughly equivalent to walking 5 miles or 8 kilometres and is a great goal to strive for if we are measuring our steps.

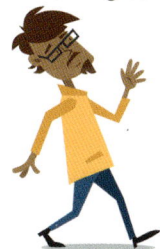

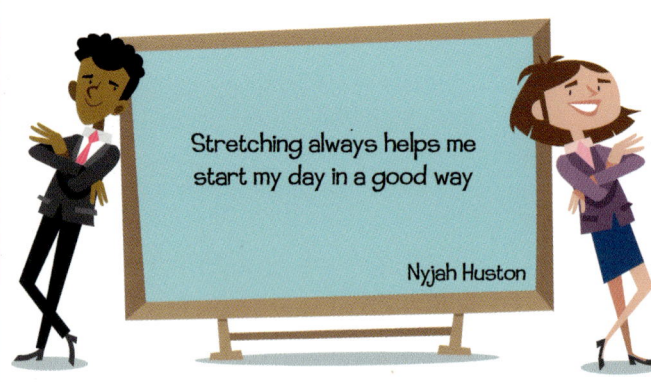

Get stretching

Stretching is an excellent mood-boosting activity and stretching in the morning helps increase our blood flow and prepares our bodies for the day ahead. When we find ourselves sitting in one place for a prolonged period it is good to get into the habit of standing up every thirty minutes and stretching.

Regular stretching helps keep our muscles flexible, strong and healthy, and we need that flexibility to maintain a range of motion in our joints. Even if we only do it for a few minutes, it will make us feel great and can be uplifting and energising.

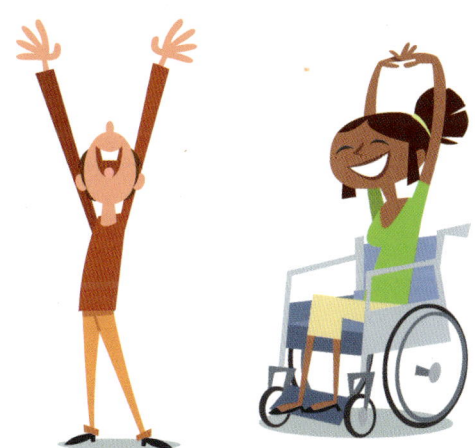

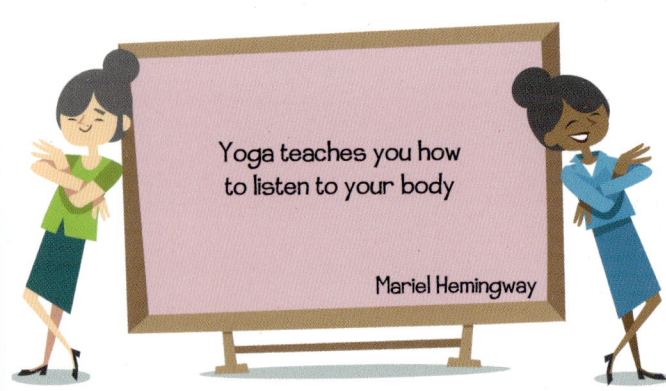

Get into yoga

Yoga is a form of exercise that evolved from ancient India thousands of years ago. The main components of yoga are postures and a series of movements that are designed to increase strength, flexibility and breathing. Regular practice of yoga can support many health benefits, including increased cardiovascular fitness and improved muscular strength. Yoga is also a renowned antidote to stress and can promote better sleep.

There are many types of yoga so it is worth exploring which one is the most appropriate depending on your age, health and mobility. Desk yoga has become increasingly popular and is well worth exploring. Hatha and Yin yoga tend to be recommended for yoga beginners as they both take a slower pace than some of the other styles.

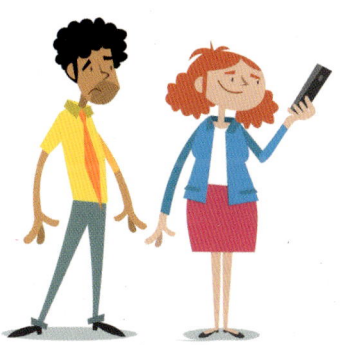

Get into Pilates

Pilates is a type of mind-body exercise developed in the early 20th century by a German physical trainer called Joseph Pilates. It is made up of simple, repetitive exercises to create muscular exertion. Pilates is a functional form of fitness that aims to enhance our mobility by integrating and working the four S's: Strength, Stamina, Stretch and Stability.

The main aim of Pilates is to increase muscle strength and tone, particularly in our abdominal muscles, lower back, hips and buttocks because these are the core muscles of our bodies.

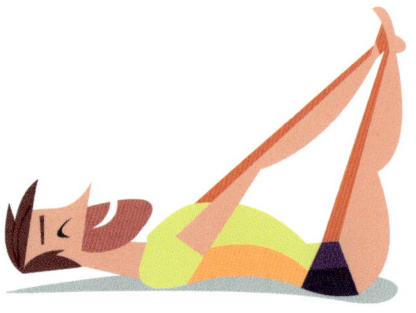

Get into strength training

Strength training is any form of exercise involving weights or resistance and is aimed at building strength in our muscles and protecting our bones and joints. Examples of muscle-strengthening activities include the following:

- ✔ Lifting weights
- ✔ Working with resistance bands
- ✔ Climbing stairs
- ✔ Hill walking
- ✔ Cycling
- ✔ Push-ups
- ✔ Sit-ups
- ✔ Squats

NB – To avoid injury if you are not sure whether you are doing a particular exercise correctly, ask a registered fitness professional, gym instructor or exercise physiologist for help.

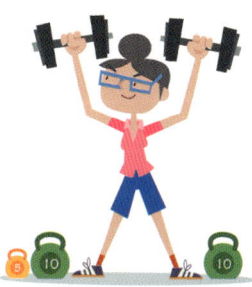

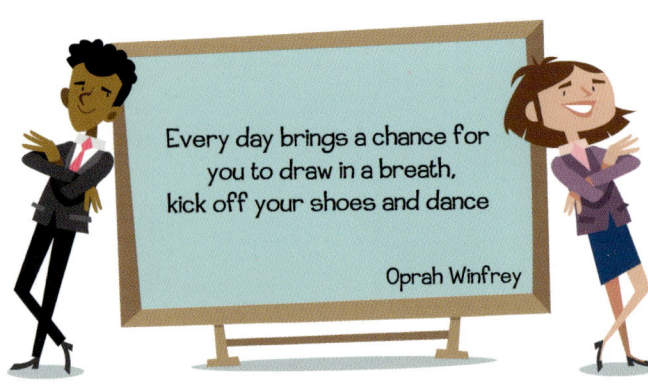

Get into dancing

Dancing is a great way to get moving and let go of tension and stress. It helps us to physically express ourselves and when we feel free, our bodies release happy hormones like dopamine. This hormone helps lift our mood and can reduce anxiety and depression.

Dancing can also significantly improve our strength and flexibility, aerobic power, lower body muscle endurance, balance and agility. Dance is also a great vehicle for social connection and bringing people together in a joyful way and there are lots of different dance classes available. Also, putting on some of our favourite music and dancing about for a few minutes can be a great energiser and stress reliever.

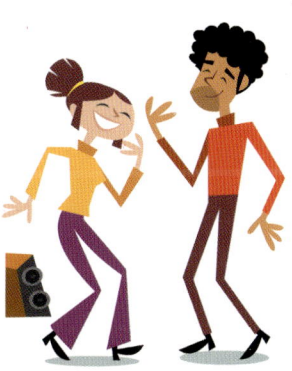

Get into sport

Getting moving by participating in a sport can be a thoroughly enjoyable way to stay active, challenge ourselves and build connections with other people. Team sports, in particular, can provide opportunities to develop useful life skills including effective communication, teamwork and collaboration.

According to the World Sports Encyclopaedia, there are 8,000 indigenous sports and sporting games played worldwide so there are lots to choose from! Even if we don't want to actually participate in a sport, we can join in as a supportive spectator. This will get us moving about and clapping and cheering, which will stimulate our senses and lift our mood.

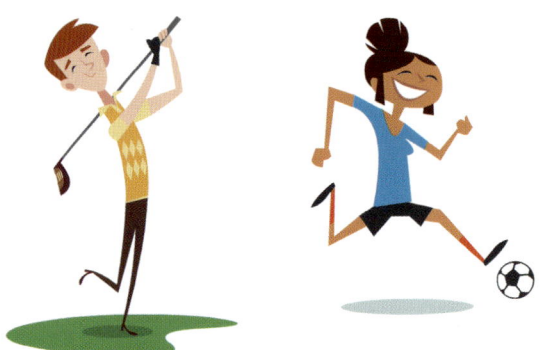

Get into swimming

One of the biggest benefits of swimming is that it's a low impact, full body workout that helps improve our heart health and muscle strength. Swimming tends to be less taxing on our joints and can be a great alternative for people with osteoarthritis or who are getting older. Swimming is an excellent way to work our entire bodies and cardiovascular systems and, according to research, swimming can burn almost as many calories as running.

There are various strokes we can use to add variety to our swimming workout and each one focuses on different muscle groups, and the water provides a gentle resistance. Swimming is a particularly good way to relax our bodies and reduce anxiety. 'Wild swimming', which is about immersing ourselves in natural water outside, is particularly good for our mental health.

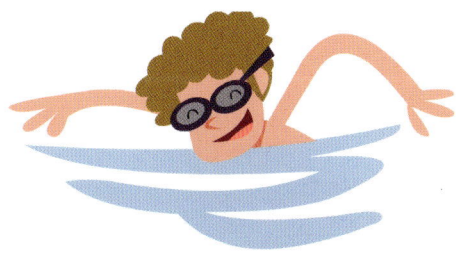

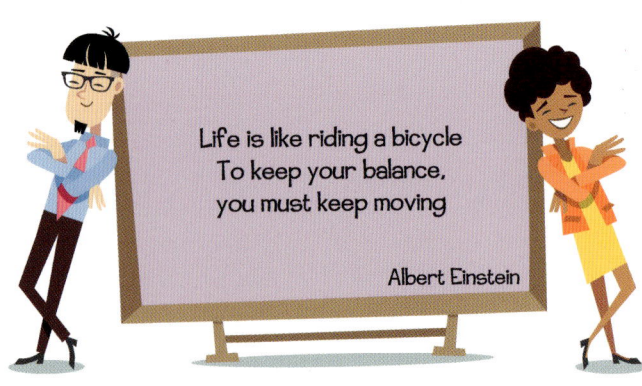

Get into cycling

Cycling is mainly an aerobic activity which can be especially good for our mental health, as well as giving our heart, blood vessels and lungs a really good workout. When we ride a bicycle we tend to breathe more deeply, perspire and experience increased body temperature, which can help to improve our overall fitness level.

By putting in consistent effort, we will notice an improvement in our aerobic capacity and this will help us to cycle for longer or on more intense rides. Also, cycling doesn't release harmful emissions that pollute the atmosphere, so when we choose to cycle rather than drive it positively supports the environment.

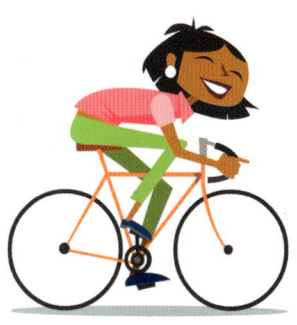

Get into running

Running is a popular form of physical activity and is a great way of exercising because it doesn't cost a lot to take part and we can run at any time that suits us. Some people choose to participate in fun runs, athletics races or marathons and it is a great way to support charity.

The difference between running and jogging is all about intensity – running is faster, which demands more effort from the heart, lungs and muscles, and requires a higher level of overall fitness than jogging. Both running and jogging are excellent forms of aerobic exercise. It is important, however, that we are aware of what suits us best and a gentle jog may be more appropriate so that we don't overstretch ourselves.

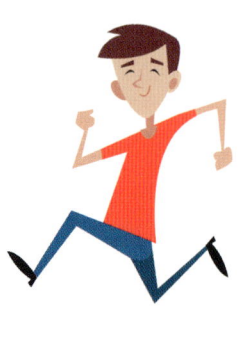

Get into rebounding

Rebounding is a type of elastically leveraged low-impact exercise and usually takes place on a rebounder which is a mini trampoline. Rebounding can revitalise the whole body in minutes by stimulating circulation and boosting oxygen levels. The act of rebounding works every muscle and is a total body workout which improves our muscle-to-fat ratio.

Jumping boosts our metabolism and improves our resting metabolic rate so we can burn calories long after our workout. Rebounding is gaining popularity because it is gentle on the joints and helps us to work our cardiovascular systems without taxing our bodies too much.

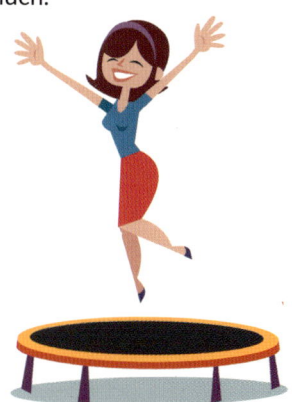

Get into nature

Moving about through nature can boost our mental health and contribute to our physical wellbeing by reducing blood pressure, regulating heart rate, easing muscle tension and managing stress levels. The natural world is the foundation of our health, wellbeing and prosperity and exposure to nature is beneficial for all of us as human beings.

There are so many ways that we can bring nature into our everyday life from exercising in the fresh air, gardening, exploring green spaces, wild water swimming or going for a bike ride. Any way that we can connect with nature will have a positive impact on our overall health and wellbeing.

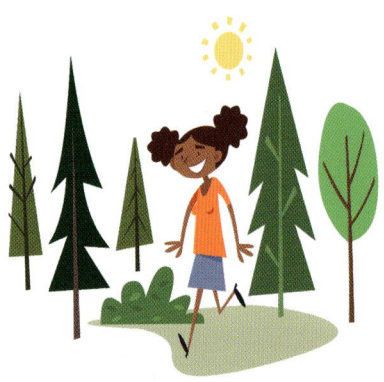

Get into gardening

Gardening is a wonderful experience that exposes us directly to the work of nature as we watch the natural world flourish. It has also been proven to improve mood, manage feelings of anxiety and depression as well as reduce stress levels.

Gardening is also a great way to get fit with digging and shovelling coming top of the list for burning the most calories and mowing and weeding not too far behind. Even if we don't have our own garden there are plenty of opportunities in the wider community to get involved by volunteering, supporting an elderly neighbour or applying for an allotment.

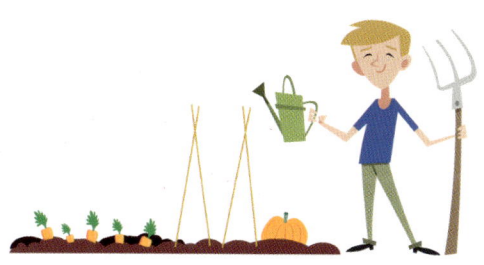

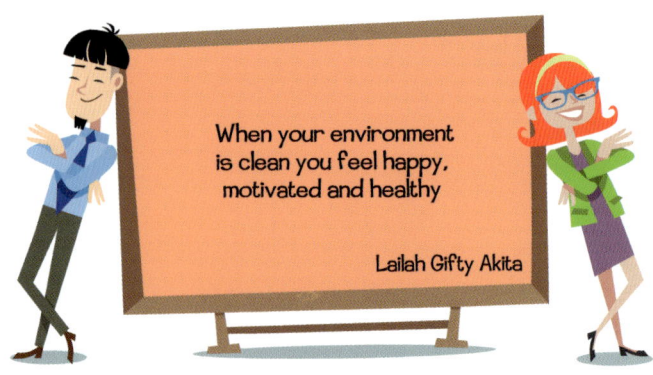

Get into housework

Housework is more than just cleaning because it involves mobility and stretching. Any physical movements carried out during housework, such as lifting, bending, squatting and reaching overhead, are all movements we may well perform during a strength training workout. Activities like vacuuming, scrubbing and lifting all require energy and when we are focused on a particular household task we may not even notice that we are exercising.

According to various experts, about an hour of intensive cleaning could be roughly equivalent to a 20-minute low-impact workout. Also, the physical activity of cleaning combined with the result of a cleaner home can be great for our mental health as it helps to reduce stress and provides us with a sense of achievement.

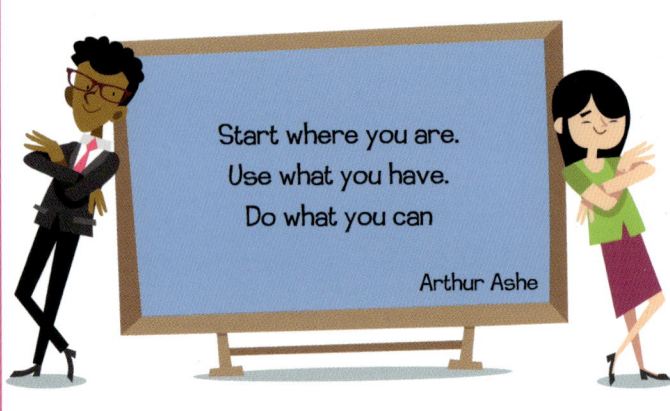

Summary

When we get moving we will feel so much better about ourselves and this will have a big impact on our mental health and overall wellbeing. Physical activity is a primary drive for us as human beings and movement is essential for thriving in life.

Trying to do too much too soon can be overwhelming and disheartening. It is better to make small adjustments such as consciously increasing our daily steps or active minutes and build up gradually. Making incidental movement part of our daily routine and reminding ourselves and each other to move about whenever we get the opportunity is a great place to begin. Get healthy, get happy, get moving!

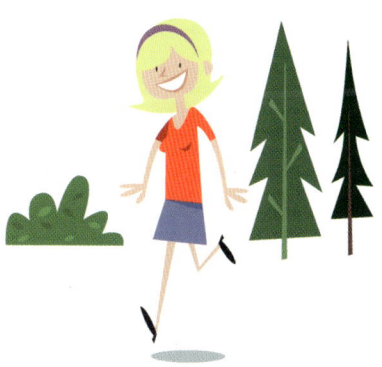

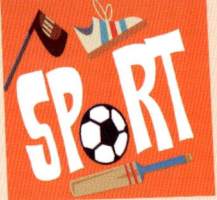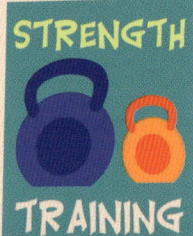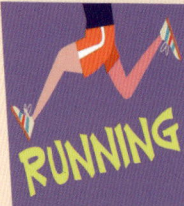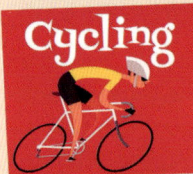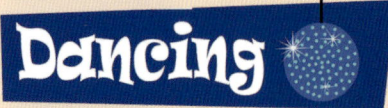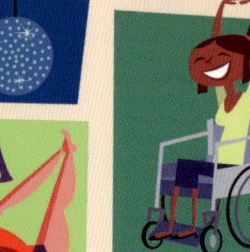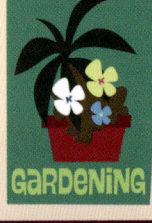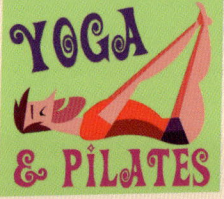